Meditation and Fasting Combined

A Powerful Healer

Joanna Aphiah

Meditation and Fasting Combined: A Powerful Healer by Joanna Aphiah.

Published by Kwizbud Publishing House, 204C Chestnut Crossing Dr.,Newark 19713, New Jersey, U.S.A.

Books@kwizbud.com

ISBN: 9781099513916

Table of Contents

Preface

Meditation and Fasting Combined: A Powerful Healer is two books in one. Or maybe I should say that most authors have always discussed and written about both of these practices as separate subjects; when indeed they are interconnected and have very potent efficacy if combined. If you are presently practicing either or both, kudos to you. However, to those who, for one reason or the other have been putting off commencing meditation and fasting; I have a few words, I love you to contemplate:

Make time each day for quiet and reflection. Our most exceptional creativity comes when we quiet our mind with reflection or meditation. Visualize your ideal life in detail and live it mentally day in and day out. Feel your perfect life like you already have it. Be open-minded. Our prejudices can keep us stuck. Don't engage in judgment or gossip. It serves zero purposes.

Finally, realize most things are neutral by nature. We make them either positive or negative. Choose the positive whenever required.

Be careful over nothing, but in everything by prayer and supplication with thanksgiving, let your requests be made known unto God.

And the peace of God, which exceeds all understanding, will keep your hearts and minds through Christ Jesus.

Finally, beloved, what so ever things are right, what so ever things are honest, what so ever things are just, what so ever things are pure, what so ever things are lovely, what so ever things are of good report; if there be any virtue, and if there be any praise, think on these things.

Joanna Aphiah

"Our scientific power has exceeded our spiritual power. We have guided missiles and misguided men."

– Dr. Martin Luther King Jr

1
Introduction

Meditation is to the mind or subconscious what fitness is to the body. The concept of fasting, which is the willful abstinence from food, drink, or both for some time, is more familiar to most of us than meditation.

When eating, you feed the body, whereas in meditation, you give food and nutrients to the mind and soul. Make out time daily for reflection and calm. Your highest creativity is born when you can shut out all external influences from your mind with meditation or reflection. Build your ideal life in detail and live it mentally daily. Visualize your perfect life as if you already have it and before long you will.

Anxiety and stress trigger more food consumption and is known to be the significant driver in alcoholism and obesity. Most alcoholics believe that the more alcohol they take will help them overcome, or at least forget, the stress they face daily. While a study on obese people had more than 90% of those interviewed stating that they chew or nibble on food all day long to overcome anxiety or stressful conditions such as after losing a partner in a relationship. As you read on, you will learn that anxiety and stress can be treated independently by either meditation or fasting. However, if you believe your particular case of stress is not responding to treatment or response is too slow using either meditation or fasting, then it is time to apply the combination of meditation and fasting for immediate treatment.

If you are addicted to alcohol or know someone who is, I will implore you to grab a copy of the book: "*Sober Forever: Overcoming Addiction and the Things I Drank to Forget*"

Most if not all of the religion of the world, has for over two thousand years, recognized the significance of fasting to our general well being, whether spiritual or physical. Jesus Christ despite His divinity and many exhibited miracles, in Matthew 17.21 made us understand that combining two virtues to deal with an issue was sure to yield anticipated result rather than tackling the problem with a single approach. In more recent times, within the last ten years, there has been increasing interest in the impact of fasting in the health sector. Intermittent fasting with improved diet has been successfully used in recent times to reverse diabetes, and people formerly living with diabetes have for about ten years lived without their medication and are in total remission of diabetes. Details of how to reverse diabetes and manage your health so that you stay free of medications for the rest of your life is covered in two books: "Reversing Diabetes: The Herbal Medicine Approach" and "*Maintaining Reversed Diabetes: Herbal Remedies to Avoid Relapse*."

1.1 Demystifying Meditation

First let's demystify meditation by saying that, it is not about transforming you into a better person or a new person; neither is it about trying to turn off your feelings or thoughts though that is incidental in the process. It's about increasing your level of awareness and growing a holistic sense of perspective. You will learn to observe things or events without judgment. And then, you shall start to gain a much better understanding of these things.

Practicing meditation is like practicing any other skill. You can relate it to exercising a muscle that you've never worked on before. It takes regular practice to get the result. And the learning process is more relaxed and better structured if you have a coach or mentor. Of course, that is where this book comes in.

Also, never beat yourself over your inability to have a perfect meditation. It is the nature of your mind to wander. That is part of the meditation exercise. What is more important is to meditate regularly. You are already winning just by showing up for practice irrespective of how the meditation eventually goes. It will take consistent practice and some time to get comfortable with your mind. Here the journey is more important than how fast you arrive at the destination. There might be hitches along the path, but that's part of meditation. Keep practicing.

1.2 Is Fasting Harmful?

The thought of fasting is quite frightening, but it is straightforward to get started. Whether you or a friend or a family member is interested in beginning water fasting, juice cleansing, detox or alternate fasting which is a type of intermittent fasting, then this book is going to be your complete reference. It is going to provide you most, if not all; you need to know to get started with alternate fasting. And there are guidelines to take care of some little intricacies that you need to pay attention to and this book will tackle those in details. We shall also study the spiritual essence of fasting if any. So we're going to cover several different things in this book, and I will quickly do an overview so that you have a solid idea of what we shall be covering.

So, we will talk about what is alternate fasting and why you shouldn't worry about its cons. We will look at the health and spiritual benefits, Fat loss, and some muscle gain.

Intermittent fasting is an eating plan, as such should not be seen as a diet. So, in essence, what you desire is to have a fixed time in which you are fasting or abstaining from food and also a specific period in which you consume all of your food and calories requirement. You're going for an elongated period without eating. And then you're going into, your "fed window," a period when you are eating. Someone is assumed to be fasting if it is over eight to twelve hours since they had their last meal. However, you have to understand fasting is not the same as 'shifting your meal time' or skipping breakfast and then having to eat 'brunch' which is having a breakfast meal together with a launch meal at launch time. Fasting is abstinence. There has to be that act of entirely missing a meal or more on a particular day, and you don't replace it later. It is gone once you skip it at its appropriate time. But if you eat the equivalent of your regular three meals during your eating window, then you haven't fasted. There has to be apparent abstinence from eating and drinking compared to your typical daily pattern, when not fasting.

Though it is human nature for us to worry; one of the biggest problems that people have with fasting is that they tend to complicate things. So you need to keep it very, very simple. However, there is plenty of different intricacies in between, but for all intents and purposes, intermittent fasting is just not eating for some time and then making-up for your calories later.

2
Spiritual, Health & Physical Benefits

2.1 Meditation Benefits

The person who meditates regularly will develop the capacity to focus, on whatever he chooses to work on, without distraction. They can achieve remarkable results. That is possible because they have strengthened their mental state and learned to stabilize their mental health through meditation regularly.

Let's discuss seven excellent benefits of daily meditation, especially for those who live in the cities around our stress-filled world:

2.1.1 Stress Reduction, Cortisol imbalance

Psychologists and Doctors often recommend that you try meditation when you're dealing with anxiety or stress. When it comes to stress relief, many people think you should deal with your stress by simply avoiding the things that worry you, as such you often hear friends and family advising you to "stop worrying." But mental and physical stress can come from just about anywhere. It can come from our friends and family, our finances or our jobs so it may not be something that you can avoid. But by learning how to meditate, you can keep the source of stress while significantly reducing the impact of stress and thus having to make any changes to your lifestyle. But you might be saying "how can sitting in silence for 10 or 15 minutes have such a beneficial effect on your life when we're stressed about passing your professional examinations or repaying mortgage loans.

The hormone "cortisol" produced by our bodies is responsible for most of the adverse side effects associated with anxiety and stress. Cortisol can disrupt your sleep, increase your blood pressure, and impair your memory, all of which can make you feel unmotivated and fatigued. Cortisol imbalance can lead to chronic anxiety and depression, which can bring your productive lifestyle to a catastrophic halt. Luckily at 2013 study found that mindfulness meditation effectively took care of stress by decreasing the adverse side effects of cortisol production. A second study which examined over one thousand participants found that regular meditation lowers stress more than almost all single psychological or medical treatment in the market. From both studies, the results were consistent for people of all experience levels and ages.

2.1.2 Self-Confidence Booster

Almost everyone struggles with low self-esteem or Self-confidence, daily. In a world filled with critics and bullies, it can be challenging to maintain and develop a lasting positive self-image. Without it, you may be battling daily to avoid another episode of depression. If this seems like you, mindfulness meditation can help you develop the type of self-esteem that won't collapse the next time something doesn't go as planned. Research commissioned in 2005, showed that the development of a more profound understanding through meditation often results in the growth of self-esteem. In this study, researchers had a group of individuals diagnosed with breast cancer to practice mindfulness meditation for 12 weeks at the start of the study each participant was tested and showed shallow levels of self-esteem, but after 12 weeks of meditation, the entire group showed remarkable improvements notwithstanding their chronic illness. Mindfulness meditation doesn't only help you build self-esteem; it's even more relevant at stopping your self-esteem from dropping at the slightest impact. Negative thoughts discourage you from doing the things that make you happy. When you encounter failure or social rejection you may start having cyclical negative thoughts which could quickly destroy all of the self-esteem that you previously built up. So it's just too necessary to address them before they get out of hand. Mindfulness meditation is a fantastic way to do just that because it presents you the opportunity to point your attention to the negative thoughts or habits and find ways to correct them.

2.1.3 Overcome Depression, Avoid Brooding

For some years now, mindfulness meditation has been used as a therapy for individuals having depression. Meditation promotes a more stable emotional mindset by lessening the presence of harmful behaviors; while also decreasing the production of chemicals in our brains, which are linked with depression. For example, it is normal amongst individuals with depression to display Brooding which permit negative emotions like sadness anger and self-criticism to manifest for a long while.

Research by the University of Exeter studied the behavior of two groups of people who were recovering from depression'; the first group used only prescriptions for depression, while the second group practiced mindfulness meditation, at least once daily, in addition to the drugs. The investigators found that about half of the group being treated only on drugs ended up relapsing because of unhealthy behaviors like brooding which prevented the pills from doing its job. Whereas for the second group, those practicing meditation in conjunction with the prescription medicine were far less likely to relapse to the absence of brooding behaviors. Which is to say, if you're battling to control your emotions and improve your mental health; mindfulness meditation is a safe and effective way to stop depression at an early stage.

2.1.4 Improved Sleep

Have you ever thought of how long it takes you to fall asleep at bedtime? The duration can vary from between ten to twenty minutes for your body to calm down, shut down and hibernate. Difficulty falling asleep can also be a sign of insomnia if it takes you an hour or more to fall asleep. Otherwise, it could mean you're just going to bed too early but believe it or not, over half the population are challenged with insomnia which can span anywhere from a few days to a few years. The majority tend to resort to sleeping pills, but these can have several nasty side effects including fatigue and addiction; so psychologists are now recommending meditation as a safe and healthy alternative. Meditation, before bedtime, gives your mind and your body the time to reduce stress and physically wind down according to a 2015 study. This short period of relaxation (meditation) can significantly improve the quality of your sleep even for chronic insomniacs. It can stop you from randomly waking up in the middle of the night because you're getting a better night's sleep while helping you fall asleep faster, and stay asleep longer. you'll also notice improvements in problem-solving and memory concentration which require your brain to be well-rested and sharp

2.1.5 Pain Management

The intensity of pain that you feel is often based upon your perception. By implication, if you can learn to control your state of mind, you can reduce the extent of pain you're feeling at any given time. Daily practice of mindfulness meditation is an effective way to sharpen that controlled mentality which will allow you to handle and lessen the level of pain that you're feeling. Yeah, it almost sounds superhuman but a 2011 research found that individuals who meditate daily seem to experience less pain than other people. This was determined by looking at the activity of their brains while in pain. The findings showed that the persons meditating daily, reacted far less to painful stimuli in comparison to people who had never meditated before. Then another study investigated pain tolerance with over three thousand participants struggling with chronic pain. They discovered that those participants who practice daily meditation were much better at coping with their grief. Whether you struggle with a chronic illness or the next time you get hurt, don't forget that daily meditation can potentially decrease your perception of pain

2.1.6 Expanded Memory

Though not often recognized as one of the main benefits, daily meditation can have a massive effect on the parts of our brain that process (store and recover) our memories. The best case of this was shown by a study in 2013 in which a group of researchers studied the brains of people who had never meditated versus people who meditated every day. While they found that the brains of longtime meditation practitioners were more developed in several different areas the regions linked with memory were some of the most well-known. These regions were thicker more complex and more active than their counterparts which the researchers ascribed to daily meditation this means they not only have an easier time recalling events from their long-term memory but can also store information much more efficiently. These skills are beneficial no matter who you are. So start practicing meditation to make sure you never forget your keys, your phone or other essential details of your life.

2.1.7 Improved Attention

The toughest aspect of meditation, most people say, is keeping your mind still. Your mind is used to continually flipping around thinking about your family, work and all your interest that it can be hard to focus on nothing or something simple like your breath. But by practicing this focusing, you're increasing your concentration capacity so that you can easily be clear-headed and be highly productive when you switch your mind to work. In 2007 a study tested the active skills of people before and after an eight-week course on mindfulness meditation. The research discovered that meditation significantly improved their performance and speed despite having never meditated before the eight-week course. Some other studies have proven that daily meditation can increase your focus and thus your productivity.

2.2: Fasting Benefits

Fasting has been practiced for so many centuries now, by religious and non-religious persons for various reasons and a long list of benefits. So let's briefly talk about the benefits. Let's look at a few of these reasons why we may consider fasting.

There are many benefits to fasting, and that's probably the main reason that people are attracted to alternate fasting, Physical benefits include dramatic, fat loss while maintaining muscle. And there is a multitude of verified health benefits such as your vascular function, as well that can improve your look, helps with the reversal of type 2 diabetes and increasing weight loss.

You can use alternate fasting with keto, paleo, or vegan or whatever you want.

2.2.1 cardiovascular Health

Further research carried out on a group of people fasting has shown that occasional twenty-four hour fasting can improve cardiovascular health.

2.2.2 Mental Health:

Fasting improves mood, alertness, helps control symptoms of depression and enhances feelings of well-being.

2.2.3 Weight Loss:

Fasting for periods shorter than twenty-four hours (intermittent fasting) is suitable for maintaining a lean body mass, as it is effective for weight loss in people with obesity.

2.2.4 Medical Use

Prolonged fasting from eight to seventy-two hours (depending on the person's age), usually referred to as "diagnostic fast" is conducted under observation to make possible the investigation of a health complication, usually hypoglycemia. Most people also fast as a requirement of a medical a check-up or test, such as preceding surgery or colonoscopy. Fasting is also done as part of a religious ritual.

2.2.5 Spiritual Fulfillment

Fasting is practiced in several Christian denominations and is done either individually, or collectively during specific periods of the liturgical calendar as a believer feels led by the Holy Spirit. Various Christian denominations input varying details and elements of practice into their fasting. While some observe a forty-day partial fast, referred to as "Lent Fast," to commemorate the fast done by Jesus Christ during his temptation in the desert, others abstain from food for a whole day (known as the "Black fast") until the evening and traditionally breaks the fast at sunset. Again, some denominations regard the abstinence from Meat and Milk as partial fasting.

Matthew 17:21 states, "Howbeit this kind (insanity) goeth not out but by prayer and fasting.

2.2.6 Behavior Development

Fasting helps develop good behavior and strengthens control of impulses. During the holy month of Ramadan, believers through fasting and prayers strive to purify soul and body and increase their taqwa (God-consciousness and good deeds).

2.2.7 Longevity:

Studies on fasting groups have linked regular fasting to a lower risk of disease and longevity. Persons who fast regularly live a healthier and longer life.

2.2.8 Expanded Memory:

Not eating for a day has many health benefits beyond aiding weight loss, Some evidence from a study on animals shows that fasting can help improve memory

3
Methodology

3.1 Types of meditation

1. Loving-kindness meditation:

Also known as Metta meditation, Loving-kindness meditation's goal is to nurture an attitude of kindness and love toward everything, including your enemies and even things that constitute a stress to you.

Loving-kindness meditation is designed to encourage feelings of love and compassion, for oneself and others. This type of meditation might enforce positive emotions and has been linked to reduced post-traumatic stress (PTSD), anxiety, and depression. It can help those affected by interpersonal conflict, resentment, frustration, and anger.

In most variants of this meditation, the basic strategy is to repeat a message severally, until the practitioner is engulfed with an attitude of loving kindness. For instance, while breathing deep, the practitioner opens his or her mind to receiving loving kindness. He or she then sends a message of loving kindness to specific people, to their loved ones, or the world.

2. Mindfulness meditation:

Mindfulness meditation is something people can do irrespective of their location, time, and age. For instance, while waiting in line at the grocery store, a person could calmly notice their surroundings, including the smells, sights, and sounds. A variant of mindfulness is involved in most types of meditation, such as Body scan meditation and Breath awareness meditation.

Mindfulness is a variant of meditation that urges practitioners to remain aware and present at the moment. Mindfulness encourages awareness of a person's current surroundings rather than dwelling on the past or dreading the future. There is a lack of judgment with this type of meditation. So, rather than reflecting on the frustration of a long wait, a practitioner is only expected to note the delay without judgment.

Because mindfulness is a context common to many variants of meditation, it has been extensively studied. Research has found that mindfulness can improve relationship satisfaction, lessen impulsive, emotional reactions, improve memory, improve focus, reduce fixation on negative emotions.

Some evidence suggests mindfulness may improve health. For instance, an investigation of African-American men with chronic kidney disease found that mindfulness meditation could lower blood pressure.

3. Breath awareness meditation:

Breath awareness meditation is a type of mindfulness meditation that utilizes mindful breathing.

As a variant of mindfulness meditation, breath awareness offers many of the same benefits as mindfulness, which includes greater emotional flexibility, improved concentration, and reduced anxiety.

Practitioners breathe deeply and slowly while focusing on their breaths and counting their breaths. The aim is to focus only on breathing, which in turn helps to ignore other thoughts that crip into the mind.

4. Progressive Relaxation or Body Scan Meditation:

Body scan meditation, sometimes called Progressive relaxation, is a meditation that requires people to scan their bodies for areas of tension. The aim is to identify the strain and then allow it to release.

Some variants of progressive relaxation require people to tense and then relax their muscles. Another form requires you to visualize a wave, traveling over your body to release tension.

Body scan meditation can help to develop a general feeling of relaxation and calmness. Some people use this variant of meditation to help them sleep since it steadily and slowly relaxes the body. It may also help with chronic pain.

During a progressive relaxation session, a practitioner starts at their feet, and work through the whole to their head.

5. Kundalini yoga:

Kundalini yoga is a physically active variant of meditation that combines movements with mantras and deep breathing. People usually learn from an instructor in a class. However, someone can study the poses and mantras at home through reading instruction guides or watching videos.

Similar to other variants of yoga, yoga can improve physical strength and reduce pain. It may also improve mental health.

A study in 2008 of veterans with chronic low-back pain, for instance, found that kundalini yoga increased energy, reduced pain, and improved overall mental health by reducing anxiety and depression.

6. Zen meditation:

Also called Zazen meditation, the Zen meditation is a variant of meditation culled from Buddhist practice. Most Zen practitioners study under an instructor because this kind of meditation involves specific postures and steps.

Again, this variant of meditation, despite its similarity to mindfulness meditation, requires more practice and discipline. People seeking relaxation and a new spiritual path may prefer zazen meditation.

The goal is to secure a comfortable position, focus on breathing, and mindfully observe your thoughts without judging them.

7. Transcendental Meditation:

Transcendental Meditation is a spiritual variant of meditation. Where the practitioner's goal is to transcend or rise above the person's current state of being as they stay seated and breathe slowly. Persons who practice Transcendental Meditation report both heightened mindfulness and spiritual experiences.

Practitioners focus on a mantra during a meditation session. The mantra is usually determined by a teacher, based on a complex set of factors, like the year the teacher was trained or the year the practitioner was born. An alternative, however, allows people to choose their mantra. This more modern version is not technically Transcendental Meditation, though it looks very similar.

A mantra is a repeated word or series of words. A practitioner may choose to repeat "I am healthy from head to toe" while meditating.

3.2 How to Meditate

Meditation is a simple concept to practice. For example, in mindfulness, all you need to do is bring your complete attention to the present moment by focusing exclusively on who you are and where you are. Meditation will help you stay aware, relaxed and calm. It can also reduce your anxiety while allowing you to process your thoughts rationally and clearly. The final goal of meditation is to get you in touch with your emotions and senses, giving you a deeper understanding of yourself.

1. First, you must place your body in a comfortable posture. The most recommended position for meditation is to sit cross-legged. This is because it promotes wakefulness for the mind and offers balanced support for your body. But, you can also be seated in a chair, lie down, or adopt any other similar posture. The main emphasis for meditation position is that it allows you to focus your attention on the meditation without getting distracted by your body.

2. Close your eyes and breathe out and in slowly to calm your body down and then naturally as you progress into the meditation exercise.

3. Close your eyes, then focus your attention on the spot between your eyebrows. the word for meditation, In Sanskrit, is 'dhyana' and it essentially means 'to pay attention to.' There are many meditation techniques around but what they all require is the application of attention. Do not strain your eyes but be attentive and relaxed. Aim toward the tip of your nose, if looking between your eyebrows is a strain.

3.3 How to Fast

1. Keep Fasting Duration Short

Remember, no single way to fast means that the length of your fast is up to you.

Longer fasting durations increase your risk of problems linked with fasting. This includes being unable to focus, irritability, dehydration, fainting, mood changes, hunger, and a lack of energy. As a beginner, sticking to shorter fasting periods of not more than 24 hours is the best way to avoid these identified side effects. If you want to increase your fasting duration beyond seventy-two hours, you should seek medical supervision from your doctor.

Most of the well-known regimens advise short fasting durations of between eight to twenty-four hours. Though some persons prefer to perform longer fasts of forty-eight and up to seventy-two hours.

Popular regimens include:

The 16:8 regime: This regime requires consuming food during an eight-hour window and fasting for the remaining sixteen hours daily, every day of the week.

The 5:2 regime: Requires you to restrict your calorie intake for two days per week (600 calories per day for men and 500 for women).

The 6:1 regime: This regime is like the 5:2, but it's only one day of the week that you are required to reduce your calorie intake instead of two.

"Eat Stop Eat" regime: A twenty-four hour complete fast once or twice per week.

2. Eat a Little portion on Fast Days

Generally, fasting involves the removal of some or all food and drink for a period of time, as such some fasting patterns like the 6:1 or 5:2 diet which allows you to consume up to around 25% of your calorie requirements in a day, on your fasting day, is a convenient entry-level fasting regime to the faint-hearted beginner. I do not consider nor recommend these regimes. However the 6:1 and 5:2 approach helps to eliminate most of the risks associated with fasting, such as hunger and feeling faint.

If you are intending to try fasting, but worried if you can cope, then limiting your calories so that you still eat little amounts on your fast days may be a safer option than performing a full-blown fast. Also the 6:1 and 5:2 makes fasting easier to sustain since you likely won't feel as hungry while doing this type of fasting.

3. Keep your body Hydrated.

Since you get between 20–30% of the fluid your body requires from food, quite often people get dehydrated while on a fast. Even mild dehydration can result in thirst, headaches, and fatigue, so it's vital to drink enough fluid while on a fast.

Most health authorities recommend the 8x8 rule, which implies eight-ounce glasses (around 2 liters) of fluid per day to stay hydrated. But the actual amount of liquid you need varies for individuals.

During a fast, you should consider drinking two to three liters of water per day. However, let your thirst determine when you need to drink more, so follow the promptings of your body.

4. Walk in the park or Meditate .

Once you commence fasting, you will almost immediately discover that you are faced with the difficulty of Avoiding to eat before your eating period, thus resulting in mistakenly or abruptly breaking your fast. This is usually a painful experience as it means a loss or waste of the time and effort already elapsed before the abrupt break.

There is an unwritten consensus that one such way to overcome unintentionally breaking your fast is to keep your mind busy, thus tricking it not to notice when you are hungry. So you want to engage in Activities that don't use up too much energy such as walking and meditating. You could also listen to a podcast, or read a book. Any activity that's not too strenuous and would keep your mind engaged is perfect.

5. Don't Break Fasts With a Feast

Breaking your fast with a feast is not advisable. It could leave you feeling stuffed and tired.

Because your overall calorie quota impacts your weight, consuming too many calories after a fast will reduce your calorie deficit, which you instead want to increase.

It could be tempting after a period of abstinence to celebrate by eating a large meal. So, if losing weight is one of your goals, feasting may harm your long-term goal by slowing down or reversing your weight loss.

The only way you should break a fast is to continue eating normally. For your next meal, eat the same quantity of food you would normally take if you weren't fasting. Don't eat a larger meal as if you are trying to make up for the one you skipper earlier in the day.

6. Stop Fasting If You Feel Unwell

If you are new to fasting, to keep yourself safe, you have to consider limiting your fasting durations to twenty-four hours or fewer and having a snack on hand in case you begin to feel faint or unwell.

Some signs that you should seek medical help and stop fasting include weakness or tiredness that prevents you from carrying out day to day activities, as well as unexpected feelings of discomfort and illness.

During your fast, you may feel irritable slightly hungry, and tired, but you should never feel ill. If you do become unwell or are concerned about your health, then you have to stop fasting immediately. Even Christ said in Mark 8:3, "And if I send them away fasting to their various homes, they will faint by the way, for many of them came from far." Christ, thousands of years ago, recognized this potentially dangerous side effect of fasting, but it didn't stop Jesus Christ from practicing fasting very often.

3.3.1 Precaution - Fasting May Not Be For You

"Fasting too long can be life-threatening. Don't fast, even for a short period, if you have diabetes because it can lead to unsafe spikes and dips in blood sugar."

I believe that most of us are quite familiar with this type of cliché above. So how do we go about fasting to ensure that it is safe at all times?

Fasting is healthy and recommended for most persons, however, if you have certain medical conditions or have had an eating disorder or trying to conceive, or you are pregnant or breastfeeding then fasting may not be suitable for you. Although fasting for short periods is generally considered safe; however, fasting could be dangerous if not performed correctly. As such, the following demographics should not attempt to fast without consulting their physician or a medical professional:

The Elderly and Children

Persons with low blood pressure

People having issues with blood sugar regulation or type 2 diabetes

People having a medical condition like heart disease

People who are emaciated, or malnourished

Persons experiencing anorexia or have experienced an eating disorder

Women trying to conceive

Women with a history of amenorrhea

Pregnant Women or breastfeeding mothers

People who are taking prescription medications

4
Intermittent Fasting Guide

We have, in the earlier chapters, discussed many different ways to fast. And it was subtly implied that there is no one-best-way to fast. Purpose and age of person fasting are two critical factors that determine your style and duration of fasting.

People may choose to fast for religious, dietary, or even political purposes. One popular method is intermittent fasting, in which you cycle between periods of fasting and eating. It entails not eating or drastically restricting your food intake for specific periods.

Fasting entails abstaining from eating for at least 12 hours. It might allow drinking water only (clean portable water or distilled water).

Fasting modus operandi include drinking only water for one or more days and Intermittent fasting modalities. This has included periods of water fasting, detox, and juice cleansing.

The challenge of only water fasting is the intensity of it. The body goes into detox almost immediately, which is excellent, because it leads to better inner purity; as such,

I would strongly recommend periods of water fasting. In my experience, for it to be genuinely manageable and effective, it should best be combined with plenty of quietness and meditation. For some considerable length of time, I did practice, water fasting for a whole day per week (i.e., 24 hours); usually on a Monday. So I'd water fast from Sunday evening after dinner, until Monday evening dinner. For a couple of years, this routine worked perfectly well. However, I wasn't able to do anything too intense on my fasting day.

When only water is consumed, exercise or other stressors should be avoided while plenty of rest is advised. Fasting Longer than 24 hours may need medical attention, especially if people are on medication. But there was a challenge with my weekly water fasting. It created 'spikes' where my body then had to readjust to natural living. And there would be compensation resulting in overeating on non-fasting days, with correspondent contraction in consciousness. So I needed to try something different, and that led to intermittent fasting. Which I logically inclined towards before it began to gain momentum and general acceptance.

4.1 Pre-Fast Planning

i). Eat Enough Protein

A lot of people begin fasting basically to lose weight. But you do not want to lose muscle while losing weight. So you don't want to be in a calorie deficit. Otherwise, it could cause you to lose muscle together with fat.

If you are eating little food on fast days, eating enough protein during your 'eating window will help you minimize your muscle loss during fasting and also offer other benefits, such as managing your hunger.

Some studies have shown that consuming about 30% of a meal's calories from protein can significantly reduce your appetite. Implying that, eating some protein during your eating window could help combat some side effects of fasting.

ii). Eat More of Whole Foods

A lot of people who fast, do so to improve their health, so eat Plenty of Whole Foods on Non-Fasting Days.

Healthy diets based on whole foods are associated with plenty of health benefits, such as the reduced risk of cancer, heart disease, and other chronic health issues.

So make sure your diet is healthy by choosing whole foods like fruits, eggs, fish, meat, legumes, and vegetables when you eat.

iii). Consider Supplements

You might become deficient in essential nutrients if you fast daily for extended periods. Nutrient deficiency may result due to continuously eating fewer calories, thus making it challenging to attain your nutritional needs.

For instance, persons on a weight loss diet are very likely to be deficient in several essential nutrients like calcium, vitamin B12, and iron. So, those who fast very often need to be taking multivitamin supplements to help prevent deficiencies. But it should be noted that it's always best to get your nutrients from whole foods.

iv). Perform Only Mild Exercise

Though some people can maintain their regular exercise pattern while fasting; it's best to keep your exercise to a low intensity when you start fasting

Low-intensity exercises could include mild yoga, gentle stretching, housework, and walking.

But more importantly, listen to your body, rest if exercising seems like a struggle when you are fasting.

4.2 Why Intermittent Fasting Works So Well

Eating one meal a day and fast for the rest of the day.

Eating for six or eight hours and fasting for the rest of the day. For example, starting at 10.00am and having the last meal at 6 pm or starting to eat at 11 am and having the last meal at 5 pm. The eating and fasting windows can be moved according to one's needs and routine

This way of performing fasting involves fasting for sixteen hours daily; often referred to as an "eight-hour eating window." You take your meals within an 8-hour eating duration and observe your fast for the remaining 16 hours. You repeat this process daily. During the fast, you can drink Coffee, Water, and other non-caloric beverages but solid food is not allowed.

If you intend to lose weight, then it is essential that you ensure you do not consume more than your usual quantity of food or calories during the eating periods. That is, eat the same amount of food per meal as if you weren't fasting at all.

There are incredible benefits ascribed to Intermittent fasting, which is why I recommend you practice it daily. Beverages for fasting include water, tea, coffee, and apple cider vinegar. Consuming anything that drives an insulin response such as drinks containing milk, juice, or sugar, will break your fast; so be careful what you take when fasting, especially if it is not a dry fast.

I should also add, that I generally don't eat in-between meals even though the eating window is increased to a maximum of 8 hours because the body still needs time to digest and absorb. If you continuously eat (grazing) during the eating window, you cause your body to continually produce insulin, which deposits excess body fat and contracts the consciousness.

So now I do intermittent fasting for at least sixteen hours every day and sometimes eighteen hours; with an eating window of about six hours to eight hours maximum. My eating window is usually between noon (or 10 am some days) and 6 pm. I have discovered it is beneficial NOT to eat after 6 pm daily because it allows your body sufficient time to digest the last meal before bedtime. It implies that my body requires less sleep, so I tend to arise around 4am-5am. This allows me plenty of early morning time to meditate and do some creative work. And because being able to practice this style of fasting daily for years, instead of once a week; my consciousness stays interconnected and expanded. I find it suited for divinely creative activities. It means you have enormous energy, and the days become incredibly productive.

4.3 Changing Our Response to Hunger

My advice to anyone experimenting with fasting, and moving into intermittent fasting as a lifestyle; you will need to work to change your inner feelings and impulse to hunger. You would, most times, feel empty, but rather than feeling the urge to reach for food, or to overload on food when you break your fast; work deep into the feeling of hunger. Because the sense of emptiness also brings with it a feeling of lightness, and from that, the sense of consciousness expansion and interconnectedness. It is at this point that the combination of meditation to fasting earns its relevance again! And as you combine both practices, you begin to see how interconnected they are and make the practice of the other, much more comfortable.

5
Mindfulness Meditation

This meditation type scripted after the Mindfulness-Based Stress Reduction program created in 1979 by Jon Kabat-Zinn to help eliminate chronic pain, stress, and other ailments, mindfulness training events can now be found in diverse venues ranging from prisons, to sports teams, to schools and recently, the U.S. Army adopted it to improve the resilience of their military .

Mindfulness' fame has been boosted by a growing body of research showing that it improves memory and attention, develops self-empathy, and regulation and reduces anxiety and stress. Some years ago, a study by an assistant researcher in psychiatry at Massachusetts General Hospital, assistant professor of psychology at Harvard Medical School and a neuroscientist going by the name Sara Lazar, was the first to document that mindfulness meditation can change the brain's gray matter and brain regions linked with memory, the sense of self, and regulation of emotions. Further research by Gaëlle Desbordes and Benjamin Shapero is investigating the beneficial impact of mindfulness meditation on depression.

Herbert Benson, Mind/Body Medicine Distinguished Professor of Medicine at Harvard Medical School and former director of the Benson-Henry Institute at Massachusetts General Hospital, as early as 1975, extolled the benefits of mindfulness meditation on the human body in the aspects of reduced blood pressure, heart rate, and brain activity.

About four decades ago, the 1980s precisely, it was not fashionable to say you were practicing mindfulness. The meditation style was yet to become a catchy phrase. In the mid-1980s, speaking of mindfulness in a medical context among scientists was "disreputable,"

"Gradually because of the research, it became elitist, no longer disreputable," said Fulton, a co-founder of the Institute for Meditation and Psychotherapy and lecturer in psychology in the Department of Psychiatry at Harvard medical school.

Despite the growing acceptance of mindfulness, many people still think the practice involves going into trances, taking short-naps, or emptying their minds. Beginners often struggle with difficult thoughts or emotions, fall asleep, feel uncomfortable, and become distracted or bored. Ardents recommend practicing the process in a group with a teacher.

Mindfulness is not about killing emotions or stopping thoughts, but rather, it is about noticing them without judgment. Mindfulness builds awareness and resilience to help people learn how to ride life's ups and downs and live happier and healthier lives.

5.1 Steps to Practice Mindfulness:

Appropriate Seating:

Locate a quiet space. Sit up straight, ensuring you are comfortable, on a chair or cushion,; allow your shoulders and head to rest comfortably; place your hands on the tops of your legs with upper arms at your side. Lying down is not an option to avoid the obvious.

Observe your Breath

Relax, close your eyes, and take a deep breath. Observe the contraction and expansion of your chest and the rise and fall of your belly. Go with the natural flow of your breath; you don't need to control it.

Staying focused

It is ok to notice your thoughts as they try to pull your attention away from the breathing, but don't judge the situation. Just return your focus to your breath. It is also ok to count your breaths as a way to stay focused.

Practice Daily

Daily practice will provide the most benefits. It can be ten to fifteen minutes per day. However, twenty to thirty minutes twice daily is recommended for maximum benefit.

6
What Ardents Are Saying

I have included comments by many practitioners of meditation and fasting here because it is always great learning from those already doing what you are aspiring to. So take out your pen and paper and get ready to learn not just from me the author but from practitioners all over the world. However, note that I am in no way endorsing the recommendation or opinions contained in any of the testimonies below.

Also, most of the questions or concerns raised in this section by the commentaries have been addressed by this book in other chapters.

6.1 Meditation Comments and Testimonies

Stephan T

I meditate ten minutes daily at 5 am. It is the first activity I perform daily after brushing my teeth and taking my coffee. It's been absolutely helpful; my life has immensely changed.

Anders F

For about three years, I have been practicing meditation but it was last year I began to do it daily, and I have seen a significant change in my behavior; such as a happier life, with reduced stress. And I am relaxed and just smiling all day long.

Shree R

There is a large assortment of meditation styles, each with different benefits and strengths.

Try out and evolve a style of mediation that is suited to your goals and will elevate your standard of life, even if you only have a few minutes to do it daily.

Everyone should do Meditation to improve their emotional and mental health. You can do it whenever and wherever!

Kushal S

meditation raises contentment, happiness, and productivity in life

Lara P

I am excited that you mentioned 'brooding' here. It's almost becoming so much m pervasive in this hyper-stimulated world.

Hari O

Thanks to ancient Rishis for giving humanity the knowledge of meditation.

Dan O

I feel catatonic, which is great because I would have been concerned if I wasn't feeling so catatonic. I meditated so much my mind has turned off that I may as well be dribbling and starring at the wall.

Sree T

I am so thankful for the ancient rushis the creators of this potent practice. I'm so proud to be an Indian.

Sajan S

Meditation teaches you to handle many challenges like remaining calm instead of your heart beating when in a shy or nervous situations

Benjamin H

If most people learn to meditate, just like understanding the health benefits of something familiar as taking a cold shower then obviously, multi-billion dollar businesses will go bankrupt soonest.

Shady L

Lets cut a long story short; meditation will improve your life.

Keesh M

I've been meditating for around a year now and wholeheartedly approve of all the rewards mentioned in this book. I am glad you have put this great information out for those who are still unaware of the incredible rewards and encourage them to take on the practice.

Ronin C

I use meditation for a lot of purposes, but that last one is a huge one for me. I use Reiki for healing myself, and it works perfectly. Let me also add that quartz can increase the healing as well if used in your meditations and if used with intent. The intent is important.

Kery C

I am unable to do it; my mind goes riotous.

Carmen S

Since I began meditation, my entire life has turned for a positive experience.

I feel calmer, more awareness, I enjoy every single moment and sleep better daily.

Leto E

Every morning, on a daily basis, I meditate for 1 hour while during weekends for five to fifteen minutes. I have been on this for the past one and a half years now.

I haven't seen much benefit though; depression doesn't go away forever; it only goes away entirely for some days only to relapse and hit hard again. My creativity is high, but I can't say if it is more than before. I have noticed that I am able to concentrate longer, but mostly on the things, I believe that matter. With regards to sleep; it is the same as before as I still have trouble falling asleep.

In summary, I am saying meditation does help, but it's not as fantastic as I see it being portrayed.

Alex Zandani

I need help, I have been doing a lot of meditation for the past forty-five days, and I still have negative thoughts, that gets the best part of me. At the time of commencing my meditation, things were good, but as the days went by, I felt like I was the same as I was before I began practicing meditation. Why do I feel like this?

James C

I certainly feel less stressed after meditating.

6.2 Fasting Comments and Testimonies

Donna B

Why didn't we come across this information twenty-thirty years ago? I'm fifty-five years old and just beginning to practice regular fasting. So, for you, younger ones, that already have this information, listen up, start practicing fasting, and don't wait another day! I don't need to lose weight, yet I can attest that the health benefits alone are fantastic.

Vibeke R

If you don't fast as regards the world, you won't find the kingdom. If you don't practice the Sabbath as a Sabbath, you will not see the father. God bless you

San Daz

Losing electrolytes in body fluid can cause dizziness. Similarly, when you go into ketosis, you will lose a lot of salt from urination. That's why you experience headaches. So you can drink salt water when doing any fasting. Secondly, if you are a person who is obese, then not eating for some hours will not kill you. That's the work of fat; it's an energy source to keep you well and alive when you go for long periods without food. But ketosis allows you to stay focused so you can "hunt" for more food. Eating three meals a day with snacks in between is a modern luxury. Back in you didn't have constant access to food. But we forget that our bodies haven't changed since the cavemen days.

Love P

I feel fine eating once daily and exercising twice daily. I have never experienced dizziness or any issue for me! I was 400 lbs, but I have lost 130 pounds, and I have seventy more lbs to go. I don't refer to it as fasting, though!

Joseph K

I've noticed a lot of the comments saying they are fasting and not losing or still hungry. i) Make sure you are exercising ii) make sure you're drinking enough water and iii) Make sure you're eating healthy full meals.

Bee Z

Intermittent Fasting is supposed to be for a Lifetime change and not just for a diet!

Aisha J

Please do your research! Research is essential, and these aren't dark things, there are explanations, scientific ones, and Intermittent Fasting can be altered and controlled, and YOU are in control of all these things. Like When you eat, what you eat and The calories in each meal. Nothing hidden or obscure, all explainable.

Nickie C

Human beings aren't supposed to eat food all day long. Eating a meal per day is ok! We have gotten used to bad habits such that we think what's unhealthy is normal.

Elizabeth B

I combine intermittent fasting with keto. I usually fast between sixteen to twenty hours and have either two small meals or one massive (1300 calories) meal, within my eating window, with no snacking. I lost a ton of weight! My goal is to reach 130lbs, and I am only 15 pounds away! I lost a lot of hair when I was starting; it's growing back now. Anyways, has anyone else noticed plateaus? I have to switch up my eating and fasting schedules to break my fast also. I have been on these diet plans since August 26, 2018.

Tina Marie

I re-started my weight loss. My eating window is between 5 am and 12 noon. So my fasting is from 12:30 to 6 pm. No eating after 6 pm. Initially, I tried to eat only once a day, but I couldn't sustain it. I can't help desiring that second meal.

Glam P

Alternate fasting is genuine! I'm 97,7kg today being Thursday and only a week from last Wednesday when I was still 99,8kg. Sister! I can't wait to see what I will weigh two weeks from now.

Queen G

I'm having a difficult time commencing fasting. Every time I decide this is the day I always end up mistakenly eating and ruining my fast.

Saint A

I eat my one meal at 9:30 pm as I maintain only one-hour eating window between 9.30 – 10.30pm. I eat healthy fats such as various seeds, nuts, bananas, dates, potatoes, and occasionally a burger. Fasting has been fantastic for me. I don't get hungry in the twenty-three hours of not eating. I feel fantastic and don't wake up with aches or feeling hungry. I am energized when I wake up.

Evette C

People, please research. Because research is very vital. Those are signs of electrolyte imbalance. Your minerals are low. Look into pink Himalayan salt, magnesium, vitamin c, potassium. I encourage everyone to balance their diet and be aware of their micros and macros. If you don't eat, you won't have energy. Research minerals and body composition. Continued success. The same discipline you use to fast may be the same discipline to eat more frequently and balanced. Continued success, but if you are not eating the same, your metabolism is probably off, and your fluid balance is shifting.

Chioma C

The loss of appetite is actual. Personally, I have experienced it as I have been doing Intermittent fasting for some time now; and I am glad that my desire for food has significantly reduced (because I had issues with increased appetite in the past), I feel I am in control of my hunger now. We are all responsible adults, and you don't want to go about starving your body, so here is a solution: Prepare your well balanced meals and snacks for a week ahead, so that during your eating window daily, whether you're hungry or not you ensure that you hit your calorie target before the window is over.

Jay S

I came by various contributors advocating intermittent fasting maybe six to seven months ago! I'm 61 and weighing up to 252! I decided to try fasting 16/8 and lost 20 pounds in just a couple of months! To go further, losing another 15-20 pounds, I reduced my eating window to 4-5 hours, ie, from 11 am to 4 pm and reduced my weight without a struggle! I go off for a day or two depending on how I feel during friends' birthdays or holidays where I might drink something knowing I'll end up putting back a few pounds! I have had some side effects; my appetite can disappear occasionally, and a little dizzy, but to me, that's a good thing! I take plenty of water, green tea, and coffee! It doesn't hurt to stop meals you don't need! My doctor is so happy about my results so far! My blood pressure is down, and my weight fluctuates between 210 and 215 pounds depending on if I stick to my fasting program or not! I am now an advocate to friends and relatives all the time; including business colleagues who see the difference so I couldn't be happier for the time being!

Marie B

I agree loss of appetite is one of the side effects which can result in anorexia, and another one for me was insomnia, ie, lack off sleep. But it's still worth it. I lost a lot of weight easily and very fast too. The feeling of being able to grab any jeans and fit into perfectly is highly rewarding.

Tuco E

The first three to four days are usually the most difficult for most people. During this period, your body is still detoxing from excess amounts of sugar we eat in the past. Loss of appetite is natural and expected.

Nagutama K

I stopped fasting over the holidays, and I put on some weight, around 2 kilos. So I am want to begin fasting again. But I lack the energy to workout. Ufff, maybe I am eating too little? But I think, my stomach got smaller, internally. I think so because i get full very fast with a small amount of food intake. If I try to force myself to consume more food later, I feel like I am going to burst. What I love about intermittent fasting is that I have so much free time, is like I don't have to be disturbed about food.

Darren C

And this is why you don't do something just because you heard it was good to lose weight without doing some personal research yourself. Your peculiar eating habits may see you reverting to your previous ways. You still think eating three times daily is "customary?" It is only usual in modern times due to the sheer amount of food.

Your putting on weight is due to, you are eating at the wrong times and most probably eating the former foods that caused you to gain weight in the first instant. What you did was retrain your body to eat at different times. The dizziness and fatigue are most likely due to electrolyte imbalances.

Intermittent fasting is NOT a diet. It is supposed to be a way of eating which accomplishes more than just weight loss. Your body can heal itself of many ailments, using intermittent fasting. The only dark side to alternate fasting is how it is still perceived by the world.

To my exciting experience. I'm on day 8 of fasting and presently 426lbs in weight. I am combining intermittent fasting and ketogenic eating habits. I don't feel hungry. I used to be on Adipex years ago, and this compares to taking it.

I'm fully energized, so I go for brisk walks in my fasting state. I don't eat high carbs, bread, and sweets or whatsoever. If I want to, I Eat between 4 pm and 8 pm and nothing after. This is working for me except inadequate sleep, but I must get on my potassium and magnesium, based on my research. I'm logging everything with fasting app ZERO, MyFitnessPal, and on Instagram.

I began my fast at 11 pm (February 12), and I'm currently at 320 pounds after eight days, I'll do intermittent fasting for a month combined with daily exercise.

Kayla R

I am struggling to lose weight and need a friend to assist me on this journey. I am twenty-six years of age and a mother of three. I weigh 250 pounds presently. I have been obese all my life and battled losing weight all these years. I hope it goes well this time.

Carmen D

@Kayla R you can do it. have faith and believe in yourself weight loss is more about your mental journey than your physical activities.

Christopher F

Dasean W, good luck on your journey, but one thing I want to tell you.

I 've been overweight in the past, I tried to diet a couple of times, and I lost weight but took it back. I finally found a way to get lean.

To cut down your weight, you seriously need to change your compartment.

Doing exercise is excellent, but start by looking at what you eat.

Intermittent fasting is a great tool, but you still need to watch what you put in your stomach afterward.

Start with some sport right away, then slowly with time, decrease, if not able, totally cut-off everything with too much sugar.

Sugar became my enemy number one. Once you feel a bit better with yourself, it gives you the energy to go a step further. Eat less saturated oil, less salt. Stop patronizing fast foods. Increase your sporting activities as you feel better and leaner. In one word, do it step by step but never look back.

And for me, instead of eating chicken and pasta, I will add fibers to it while decreasing the quantity of pasta(glucides) and good oil is ten times better for your health. Also slowly stop every ketchup and its like. Sugar is everywhere. So beware. And stop deceiving yourself with cliché like, " I'm about to do a big workout so I 'll drink an energy drink.". No, you have much more energy without taking that poison.

Carla C

I'm super confused about what to eat as a vegan. Could you do a book for Vegans who do Intermitting fasting?

Hazel M

Very helpful. I think I will start tomorrow, but I only want to reduce my waist size, which is presently 31 inches. My weight is alright I guess, it is 116 pounds. I want to try fasting. Good luck to everyone currently doing intermittent fasting too.

Erin G.

I can't workout without eating, as I feel like fainting. What is your advice to people with hypoglycemia who want to start fasting?

Shrestha S

Can protein shake be taken before starting your fast?

Eamador G

Is it alright to drink any natural tea when I am fasting? Like lemon tea or green tea, etc.? What of herbal tea? Without any sweeteners, of course?

Rebecca C

I thought 20/4 fast wouldn't be that difficult, but oh man I was wrong. So I decided to try 16/8 instead before I give up too quickly.

Anne F

I started 16/8, but by the next day, I went to 20/4 and have stayed here.

Francis D

I am doing 16/8 fasting; I eat a lot of fiber before I start fasting.

Do not eat carbs with fat to break the fast it causes insulin to open cells and let fat in which is not good. I Workout and stay hydrated drinking tea or black coffee during fasting, which helps me burn more fat, especially in the muscles. The longer I fast, the smarter my brain is. Fasting helps me to become more focused.

Women's bodies send more hunger signals than that of men. Intermittent fasting helps with building more muscles compared to when eating normally or not fasting. Same as with drinks, if the supplements have calories or carb, they break the fast. Alcohol is toxic, and besides making fat to burn less effectively, it causes the liver not to function well.

Paralee W.

Great book. Lots of information and it's nice to know you have more out there. Perhaps you cover these questions in those books, but I thought I should ask:

1) If my eating window is noon to 8 pm, should I have lunch at 2 pm, a fruit or nuts snack at 4:30 PM and dinner at 8:00 PM? Or can I eat any number of times and at any time without a daily pattern?

2) due to family and work demands, I can only workout immediately after work and before going home, so I usually get to the gym by 5:00

pm. So which is better, to exercise in the middle of the fast instead of in the middle of your eating sessions?

3) is it ok to have a cheat day, like on the weekends? I believe I won't need them when I get used to the fasting, but sometimes during lazy weekends I, can't help having a hearty breakfast. Thanks!

Song B

The most significant benefit I got from alternate fasting was my appetite getting so low. I can't tell how it happened, but I would feel my stomach get full, and I know I have had enough food. Fasting has changed my eating habits, and my life is looking great.

Jaharii A.

I had the best cycle ever on this cleanse! It was amazing. I felt like I could just float and dance. I was in such a great mood! The stress from college was killing my body and diet at the time and the fast really gave me a whole new release. Enjoy your life

Mcgrable D

Keep it simple & easy.

Don't eat anything in sixteen hours (includes your sleeping time) then eat some healthy food within the next eight hours.

During the "none eating hours" drink water, black coffee, or tea only without adding any cream or sugar at all. no diet soda, diet coke, or whatever else except those three drinks earlier mentioned. People would always give excuses that it's alright to add just a little of the forbidden items like having a cheat day. But if that's the plan, don't waste your time in starting the fasting at all.

Stick to your program and never give up to see fantastic results. That's it. And trust me, it works 100%.

Aspasia O.

Personally, I have tried all of the above methods, and at present, I do intermittent fasting most times. If for any reason, on a given day, my eating window becomes more extended, then I will make sure, that I return to the recommended eating plan again the next day. I find this way of long term fasting suitable for my schedule and full of energy, vibrant, and feeling healthy. Intermittent fasting is also a way to tame cravings as and when they arise and to process corresponding challenging emotions.

I also have a diet, which is entirely plant-based and mostly whole foods, as such, the discomfort that most people, often experience with fasting programs like excessive tiredness, dizziness, headaches, etc. is very very mild in my case. Experts have reported that the more sugar, salt oil, refined carbs, and animal-based diet we consume, the more withdrawal symptoms of illness and feeling unwell. Same applies with the response to medications between persons who consume animal or meat-based food compared to persons consuming plant diet. Therefore, to begin fasting for the very first time, one may need to first start a detox or cleansing program by eliminating unwholesome foods, earlier listed, and feeding the body with vibrant plants foods for a while.

Vimal V.

The information is invaluable. I had attempted juice fasting, and water fasting and the former is a bit more practical. I have had beautiful expansion while fasting and meditating or listening to music. The last time I did a water fast, I was filled with emptiness, frustration, and hunger. So it has been a few months since I did fasting for the same reason. When next I fast, I tend to eat fast foods when breaking my fast to make up for the intensity. For several weeks now, my mind feels a bit clogged, making me feel the urge to fast. The intermittent fasting makes sense to me. I will be trying it in the next few days. Thank you.

Lisa W.

Most days for twelve to sixteen hours, I try to do intermittent dry fast (no eating or drinking). Since this year, when I became aware of the benefits, I have performed four twenty-four-hour dry fasts. The more I practise meditation, the easier it gets. I am not even drinking water. So far, being someone who loves food so much, I am impressed with my willpower, but I am still waiting for a fantastic insight into the subject.

Jen D.

Hi Aspasia, thanks for the information. The advantages of intermittent fasting and meditation are becoming more familiar, among health-conscious populations. It was fascinating to find out that intermittent fasting allows rejuvenation, integration, and a deep cleanse on so many levels. I think intermittent fasting is the best of two worlds - cleansing and eating at once. Testing and changing old patterns are involved as it could take some transformation from long-held ideas about the need for food to provide energy. For instance, there is a belief that you will need calories before you go to exercise or start your day. But instead, I have found that I feel much more energetic at the gym or through the morning when I don't eat any food. I prefer to come home and have a juice or a smoothie after I go for a walk or return from the gym.

I discovered that I savor the sense of emptiness and lightness, and when I eat, I consume far less quantity than I use to when eating on non-fasting days. There is a quicker sense of satisfaction from less, and I enjoy the idea of feeling satisfied but not full or over-filled. I recall then in my office working days we would all go to lunch and eat these large meals – you would then need to gulp vast volumes of coffee to keep the energy up in the afternoon only to observe that all the food and drink intake has lead to a significant drop in energy.

7
Herbs for Meditation and Fasting

7.1 Herbs for Meditation

Herbal medicine has been used for centuries around the world, often to treat physical ailments. Some herbs ease sore muscles and tension after practice. However, we know some herbs go beyond the physical and can address the state of mind, affecting the very state of our consciousness.

The most obvious of these are referred to as psychoactive plants. These plants quickly reach the brain and cause states of euphoria or hallucinations. But there is extensive debate regarding the effective use of these plants; most modern meditation adepts agree that they have significant limitations and might be another distraction from realizing the true self.

Below are some natural herbs that assist meditation practice. They can calm and strengthen the mind, making it easier to stay alert, become still, and enter into meditation. The herbs are:

Tulsi (Ocimum sanctum)

Tulsi, also called holy basil, is referred to as the meditation herb. In India, it is believed that the goddess Vishnu lives in it. As such, It is a sacred plant that is kept near temples and homes to sanctify and purify them. Tulsi was mentioned in two ancient texts, the Sushruta Samhita and Charaka Samhita, and is said to bring goodness, virtue, and joy. Studies have shown that it prevents increased levels of corticosterone (a byproduct of stress),. enhances cerebral circulation, and protects the brain

Brahmi (Bacopa monnieri)

Bacopa monnieri is a perennial crop. A creeping plant that is native to the wetlands of southern and Eastern India, Africa, Europe, Asia and also North, and South America. Its use in meditation is to improve concentration, joy, and contentment, perhaps because it increases circulation to the brain. It also stimulates neurotransmitters and dopamine receptors. Brahmi is very popular for its use in Ayurveda, and it is derived from Brahma, "the creator," who created the universe from his thoughts. Currently, Brahmi is being researched to ascertain its beneficial impact on Alzheimer's disease.

Gotu Kola (Centella Asiatica)

Gotu Kola with a leaf resembling the brain is sometimes referred to as the most spiritual of all herbs. It is used by yogis to develop the crown chakra. Gotu Kola is a juice for the nerve tissues and the mind, rebuilding energy reserves and nourishing the central nervous system; while helping to balance the right and left hemispheres.

Passionflower (Passiflora Incarnata)

Passionflower was so named by Spanish missionaries in Peru, who said the flower resembles the crown of thorns, associated with the crucifixion of Christ. Passionflower, which is a climbing plant also known as Maypop or Wild Apricot. It is nervine, which can increase serotonin levels, a naturally occurring chemical in the brain responsible for mood balance.

It is a mild sedative that calms the mind when it is agitated or anxious. So it has been applied for ages in the treatment of anxiety disorders and depression.

Sage (Salvia officinalis)

Sage is better known as a culinary spice but also used to balance and cleanse negativity from body and mind. A perennial subshrub that can be found in almost every part of the world was originally native to the Meditteranean region. It belongs to the mint family known as Lamiaceae. Some species are held sacred by Native Americans, Current research work on Sage is establishing its efficacy to the enhancement of cognitive function and memory and improve the mood. These qualities are essential for successful meditation.

7.2 Herbs for Fasting

We are exposed to toxins daily. So your body needs to have those toxins washed out. With the fasting herbs, your body would be able to quickly cleanse itself and give you the energy you are afraid to lose from fasting. It is usually scary starting a fast, but herbs do ease that fear.

Below are herbs that assist you in having a safe and successful fast:

It's possible to make your herbal blend. You could start small if you plan to make your blend, which you could make into a capsule for ease of storage and consumption. For a guide on how to prepare capsules to go to the appendix section.

Watermelon Juice:

You prepare this by simply blending what is left of the watermelon fruit after removing the back and seeds of the fruit.

Coconut Water:

This is also good against dehydration and should be taken with your meal during your eating window to help replenish lost electrolyte. Break a coconut fruit, collect the water inside and drink. It is as simple as that.

Peppermint is a crossbreed between spearmint and watermint. A plant indigenous to places in the Middle East and Europe, the plant is now widely spread and cultivated in various parts of the world.

This herb is useful to decrease fainting and dizziness while fasting. It is also known to calm the stomach after eating irritating foods.

8
Potency of Combining Meditation & Fasting

We have seen the various benefits of meditation and also of fasting independently. So I guess everyone can imagine the remarkable benefits that would result from combing both practices. Let me start with evidence of the spiritual benefit of combining meditation with fasting. Acts 10:30 states "And Cornelius said, four days ago I was fasting until this hour, and at the ninth hour I prayed (meditated) in my house, and, behold, a man stood before me in bright clothing." This appearance is evidence of an immediate answer to Cornelius request in his meditation while fasting.

With increased clarity, expansive awareness, and strength of Mind, karmic conditioning is felt through and moved more rapidly. When I used to do 11-12 hour meditation practice over a ten-day retreat period, I would have one small meal at 11 am, and the rest of the time I drank only water. The already intense meditation practice is intensified by The fasting, and I experienced the rapid purging of conditioning through the mind (in mental energy and dreams), through the emotional body and also the physical body(tightness, flu symptoms, pain). At the end of the tenth day, I would feel immense lightness, presence, expansiveness, and peace.

Fasting has been proven in studies to have a beneficial effect on anxiety and stress, just as studies have also shown that meditation can significantly impact on anxiety and stress. As such, when combining both meditation and fasting, it is a sure strategy to ensure that the results and intended target are attained.

Studies have shown that Fasting is effective for facilitating the unfolding and 'burning' of karmic processes, for breaking addictions and for improved mental and physical health.

There is a consensus across various 'spiritual' organizations that fasting 'burns karma.' One often experiences deeper Samadhi states and also increased sensitivity to energies when combining fasting and meditation.

8.1 How to Expand your Consciousness

If you are working toward maximum expansion of consciousness, the type of food you then eat during the day is also essential. For me, I find that a fruit smoothie breakfast is a great way to begin the eating period of the day. It's light, digests quickly, and provides blood sugars rapidly (early in the day the body is still internally rebuilding, and so best not to overload with cumbersome digestion processes). Lunchtime usually consists of a raw salad, including essential fats - such as nuts and avocados. It's when I also start to consume slightly denser proteins - lentils and chickpeas, for example. And then for the evening meal, it's usually steamed vegetables and a grain - my favorite being quinoa and millet, because they are easier to digest than rice, while also being more nutritious and alkalizing.

8.2 In a Nutshell

Fasting is very good and should be adopted as a lifestyle. While you practice fasting, please ensure you meditate twenty to thirty minutes meditation as we start the day's fasting and another twenty to thirty minutes fasting when you are about to end your fast. Repeat the same method the next day.

Once you abide in the practice of meditation and fasting combined and make it a daily lifestyle, be assured that you would enjoy extreme good health, like I do. Your body and mind will be always detoxified and supercharged to chase away illness such as cancer that conventional medicine is unable to determine its cause, let alone its cure.

You would also enjoy lots of spiritual benefits. You will desire something and you will receive it. All things shall work together for your good as you begin to yield to your intuitive mind. Remain blessd.

APPENDIX:

How to Make 5-in-1 Herbal Capsule

I will be giving you details of how to make potent herbal medicine at home in capsule form. This is to ensure that you don't end up buying plain chalk instead of the actual intended herbal remedy.

Before taking this medicine, it is strongly advised that you should have corrected your diet choice to a whole food set. Depending on your body mass index, swallow two or three capsules of this 5 in 1 herb daily after meal. Allow two (2) hours apart, as it is not recommended that you take this herbal capsule at the same time of taking other doctor prescribed drugs.

First, let's look at how to prepare medicines by placing powder forms of our herbal products into capsules for easy consumption.

You will require empty capsules to fill your powders at desired potencies, thereby avoiding tablet binders and fillers. For instance "oo" gelatin capsules should hold around 700-900 mg of most vitamin powders.

WHAT YOU WILL NEED

i)   Capping Machine: A capping machine and empty gelatin capsules. "The Cap-M-Quick" can cap 50 capsules at a time, but you have to manually join the capsule ends together whereas "The Capsule Machine" can only do

24 capsules at a time. Both machines can use either size 0 or size 00 capsules. However, 'the capsule machine' joins the capsule ends together automatically.

ii)   Milligram Scale: You need a milligram scale to weigh your powders. Note that a milligram scale with 1mg accuracy is essential for this manufacturing exercise.

iii)   Herbal powders for your blend. A filler material used to fill the unused space in your capsules that your active compound did not fill. Some suggested powders include corn starch, baking soda, glutamine, flour creatine, etc.

iv)   A pestle and mortar to thoroughly mix your herbs and filler.

v)   Empty Gel Capsules

How To Make Your Capsule Blends

For this demonstration, we will assume you are using The Capsule Machine. So load 24 empty capsules into your capsule machine and fill them with your preferred filler.

Weigh the filler powder after removing the filler from the capsule machine then to get the weight of the filler ingredient per capsule, divide the weight obtained earlier by the number of capsules.

Next, obtain the weight of your active compound per capsule by repeating the above steps.

LET'S ESTIMATE YOUR SUPPLEMENTS' RATIO:

In some cases, you will need to determine the ratio between your supplements to dose your compounds accurately. We will be mixing glutamine (the filler) with equal quantities of five herbs (Sage, Gotu kola, Passionflower, Brahmi and Tulsi) which are the active compounds. Baking soda is excellent also as a filler for anxiety remedies, as such could be used in place of glutamine.

Use the measuring cup that comes with most syrup drugs to measure equal quantities of each of Sage, Gotu kola, Passionflower, Brahmi, and Tulsi powder; then thoroughly mix all together.

Now determine how many grams of the powder of the mixed herb that is contained in one capsule. This can easily be ascertained by filling a capsule with the mixed herbs and weighing it then subtract the weight of an empty capsule.

So, to obtain the weight of mixed herbs powder required to fill 48 capsules you multiply the weight of one capsule by 24.

MIX YOUR FILLER AND YOUR ACTIVE COMPOUND

If you have pre-specified weights of the various herbs and they don't add up to the total weight that the capsule size can hold, then it becomes evident that you will need to add a filler to make up the shortfall.

But for our four in one mixed herbs, using a "oo" gelatine capsule, there wouldn't be the need for a filler. The "oo" gelatin capsule holds an average of 700-900 of powder turmeric. And we will be consuming about 200mg daily of each of the four herbs bringing the total weight of the four herbs desired to about 800mg. So we know that a mixed portion of the five herbs when filled in the capsule, will amount to our desired target of about 800mg.

Now you are set to produce your first capsules!

CAPSULE FILLER MACHINE INSTRUCTIONS:

If you have never made nootropic capsules before, following the instructions above may be intimidating.

1. To mix and accurately dose your blend, you need 5g of Gotu kola, Passionflower, Sage, Brahmi and Tulsi (red milligram scoop included), 25g of Glutamine (1/8 tsp scoop included), a digital milligram scale, and a mortar and pestle.

2. With your filler and your active ingredient appropriately mixed, can begin filling the capsules. Size oo empty capsules will be needed, plus the Capsule Machine, and your mix. Load your empty capsules into the holes. The longer halves of the capsules go in the base; the shorter halves go in the lid.

3. Set the bottom of your capsule machine on its stand and set it on a plate or flat bowl to catch any powder that spilled. Then put some of your mixes onto it and use the accompanying scraper to fill the capsules.

4. Remove the base from the stand. You can now place the lid, of the capsule machine, containing the capsule tops on the base of the device. Securely, press down to join the capsule ends together. The capsule machine base is on a rigid spring and should flatten with enough force.

5. You can now push down on the back of the lid to bring out your capsules.